MW01196189

Body Energy

*Discover The Secrets Of
The Chinese Energy Clock*

Matthew Harrigan

www.BodyEnergyBook.com

Body Energy – Discover The Secrets of The Chinese Energy Clock

First Printing, 2012

ISBN-13: 978-1482053661

ISBN-10: 1482053667

Printed in the United States of America

Contents

Introduction

"Knowing others is intelligence, knowing yourself is true wisdom. Mastering others is strength, mastering yourself is true power." – Lao Tzu

While spending several years living above my in-laws' acupuncture and herbal clinic in the 1990's I became very interested in Traditional Chinese Medicine and its mysterious methods of healing the mind and body.

While reading *Chi Kung: Cultivating Personal Energy* by James MacRitchie I became fascinated by the fact that our bodies run on energy (chi) that travels along pathways (meridians) the same way electric current runs through our homes powering appliances and electric devices. Even more fascinating to me was the fact that this chi energy flowed at specific times of day and in a pattern of movement that could be followed through each of the 12 major acupuncture meridians over a 24 hour period.

The 24-hour cycle of chi is what governs the movement of chi energy throughout the body. It begins in the lung meridian at 3am and continues for 2 hours, then moves to the colon meridian from 5am until 7am. This cycle continues for 24 hours as the chi energy energizes each of the 12 major meridians and returns to the lung meridian at 3am the next day to begin the cycle over again.

If you have blockages in your meridians (similar to a tripped fuse in your home's electrical circuit) your chi energy will not be able to "power up" that meridian and will negatively affect your health and well being. Being "in-tune" with your body and how you feel throughout the day can help you recognize and understand which of your meridians may be blocked or stagnate.

In this book I give you an overview of the 12 major meridians, what time your chi will be flowing through each meridian and individual exercises and therapies (makko-ho, chi kung, and acupressure) that you can perform to help keep your body's energy flowing smoothly and efficiently at all times.

A few years ago I was introduced to the Japanese meridian stretching therapy called Makko-ho. As soon as I saw it I knew it would be the perfect exercise to complement to the 24 hour cycle of chi.

Makko-ho is a series of deceptively simple stretches designed to help re-align your body and promote chi health by stretching your meridians.

The image below is a depiction of the six meridian stretches that make up today's Makko-ho series and within the book I have coordinated them with the meridian chi flow times so that you can either

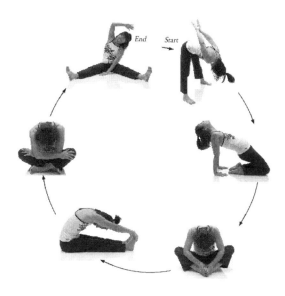

perform the entire series at once (approximately five minutes) or you can perform these postures throughout the day during the time your chi is flowing in a specific meridian.

Makko-ho stretches were the idea of shiatsu master Shizuto Massunaga's father. He had a stroke at age 42 and with one side of his body paralyzed he did not want to just give into his unfortunate fate. He decided to find a way to regain his health. He

3

obtained the idea of performing certain body postures from Buddhist prayer positions (which have been said to be performed innately by children all over the world). Over time these prayer poses developed into four main exercises and are the core of Makko-ho today. Within three years, Shizuto Massunaga's father managed to heal himself dramatically.

Performing chi enhancing exercises such as Makko-ho, chi kung, tai chi, and yoga are some of the best ways to cultivate and enhance your body energy over time.

To your health,
Matt Harrigan
www.BodyEnergyBook.com

Breath Awakens The Spirit
3am – 5am Lung Meridian Time

According to Traditional Chinese Medicine our chi (life energy) begins to flow in our lung meridian at 3am each morning.

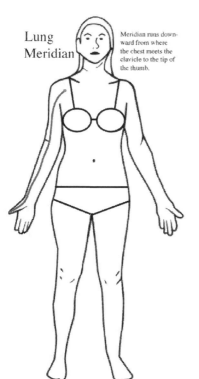

Lung Meridian

Meridian runs downward from where the chest meets the clavicle to the tip of the thumb.

Our lungs extract chi from the air we breathe and deliver it through the meridian system. Our lungs are one of our main connections to the outside world.

You should be sleeping at this time and your body should be preparing to wake up in the next few hours.

If you were following a totally natural lifestyle with no electricity or lights you would more than likely have been asleep by 8pm and would be preparing to wake at 5am. This would be a full 9 hours of restorative sleep and would keep your body and mind healthy.

However, if you find yourself awake at this time unable to return to sleep then you more than likely have an issue pertaining to the lung meridian and most likely your lungs.

It is no coincidence that most asthma attacks happen in the early morning hours between 3am and 5am. The compromised lungs of an asthmatic cannot handle the surge of chi at this time. If you or a family member continually wake up coughing at this time it is best to see your family physician or specialist for a check-up.

It is said that wearing white helps nurture our lungs and that allowing us to express emotions helps strengthen the lungs.

> *The best way to enhance your chi at this time is to be asleep.*

Lung 1 Acupressure Point:

Lung 1 acupressure point is an excellent point to massage when you experience lung difficulties. To locate Lung 1, find the depression just below your clavicle (where it meets your shoulder).

When you find that area, move in one inch on to your pectoral (chest) muscle. Use your thumb to deliver good pressure onto Lung 1 and hold for about 10 - 20 seconds then rest for 5 seconds and repeat 3 times on each side of the body.

This will help with asthma, bronchitis, and other lung ailments. In Traditional Chinese Medicine the lungs are also associated with the emotion grief. Massaging this point will help you when dealing with grief.

Lung and Colon Meridian Stretch:

This stretch is beneficial for breathing difficulties caused by anxiety, asthma, bronchitis, and fatigue from overwork.

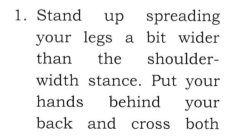

Lung 1

1. Stand up spreading your legs a bit wider than the shoulder-width stance. Put your hands behind your back and cross both

7

thumbs while the index fingers opening outside.

2. While exhaling, bend forward stretching your arms backwards and upwards.

3. Calmly inhale when your body is stretched to its limit (do not push too far) and keep this position for 10 - 30 seconds depending on how you feel. You will start to feel some contractions in your lower legs, stomach, back and arms.

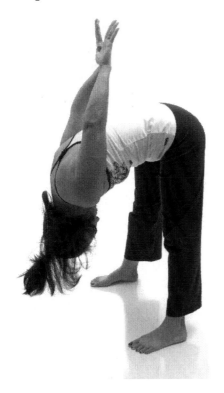

4. Now exhale slowly and steadily feel the tension loosening and relax.

5. Repeat steps 3 and 4 a few times so that your stretch in-creases but never push your body too far. Practicing this stretch will relieve many ailments that correspond to a chi imbalance in your lung and colon meridian.

The Most Important Time Of Day
5am – 7am Colon Meridian Time

If you were to visit China and wake up in the early morning you would be amazed at all the people who are up and exercising outdoors in the parks at this

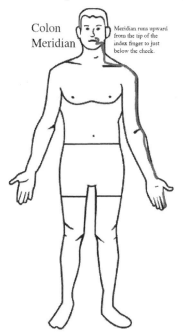

Colon Meridian

Meridian runs upward from the tip of the index finger to just below the cheek.

time. This is Colon Meridian time between 5am - 7am (also commonly referred to as Large Intestine Meridian).

I believe it is the most important part of the day in Traditional Chinese Medicine and for living in balance with nature.

The sun is rising at this time and so is your yang energy. Birds, squirrels and other animals are up early during these hours as nature intended. However, with the use of electricity, lights, television, and computers we have totally lost touch with nature. We stay up well into Gall Bladder time (11pm - 1am) and do not give our bodies a chance to complete our chi cycle properly and replenish our chi each day.

This in turn affects our ability to get up early and start the day fresh and alert. So most people start the day with a cup of coffee and make a mad dash for the office.

This will only lead to imbalanced and deficient chi in your body and eventually to illness. This is the optimal time to practice chi enhancing exercises like Chi Kung (Qigong), Tai Chi, Makko Ho (Japanese meridian stretching), Yoga or any chi enhancing exercises that you prefer and work best for you.

> *The best way to enhance your chi at this time is to exercise. Makko-Ho, Chi Kung (Qigong), Tai Chi, and Yoga exercises are excellent at this time of day.*

Large Intestine 4 Acupressure Point:

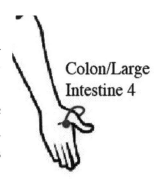

Large Intestine 4 (LI4) is a potent acupressure point. LI4 is used to relieve: headache, toothache, pain, cough, sore throat, constipation, and delayed labor. Do not use this

Colon/Large Intestine 4

point during pregnancy. LI4 is in the fleshy web on the front of your hand between your thumb and index finger about half way between the base of your index finger and your wrist. Use your thumb to press and hold this point for several slow breaths. Then alternate to opposite hand and repeat.

Governing Vessel 26 Acupressure Point:

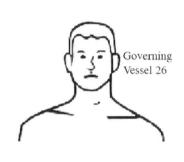

Governing Vessel (GV26) acupressure point located between the upper lip and the base of the nose about 1/3 down from the base of the nose. This point is traditionally a first-aid revival point for someone who is unconscious but is also very useful to restore mental alertness and energy.

Used in this way it can be useful at many times of the day. If you are feeling sluggish first thing in the morning you can apply pressure to this point for about one minute with the tip of your finger.

Lung and Colon Meridian Stretch:

See stretch in the previous chapter.

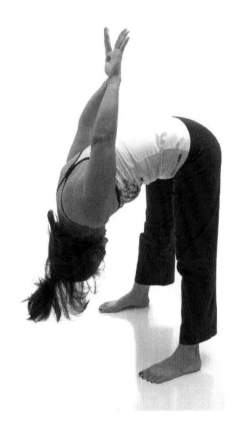

Earth Chi Nourishes
The Body
7am – 9am Stomach Meridian Time

At Stomach Meridian time (7am - 9am) the only thing you should be focusing on is nourishing your stomach meridian with a very healthy breakfast.

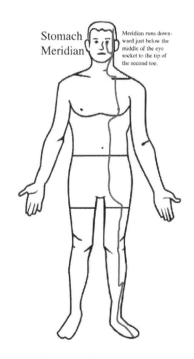

Stomach Meridian

Meridian runs downward just below the middle of the eye socket to the tip of the second toe.

Just as the lungs extracts air chi from the air we breathe the stomach extracts earth chi from the food we eat.

A very healthy breakfast will set the tone for the rest of the day and will allow your chi to flourish and build in your stomach meridian. This will pave the way for healthy chi to move to your spleen meridian, which is next at 9am - 11am. In Traditional Chinese Medicine the stomach and the spleen are a brother and sister pair with the stomach being yang and the spleen being yin. What happens in one of these meridians affects the other.

Do you think it is just a coincidence that the entire world eats breakfast between 7am - 9am in the morning? This is as nature intended but many people in Western civilization ignore this natural instinct and skip breakfast in a rush to get to work (because they stayed up into or past Triple Heater Meridian time and did not awake refreshed in Colon Meridian Time) then at work they down a cup of coffee and eat a bagel at the office. This not only depletes your stomach chi but it sets the stage for illness and disease.

According to Traditional Chinese Medicine you can support the stomach meridian by wearing yellow clothing.

> *The best way to enhance your chi at this time is to eat a healthy nourishing breakfast.*

Stomach and Spleen Meridian Stretch:

This meridian stretch helps relieve poor digestion, overeating, stiff shoulders, chronic gastric problems, and other ailments attributed to spleen chi imbalances. This stretch can be challenging so take it slow.

1. Kneel down on both knees and sit with your buttocks between your legs. Exhale and bend back-wards slowly while bringing your knees together.

2. Stretch your arms straight back and you're your shoulders to the floor. As with all stretching only do what your body will allow, do not force your stretching. Inhale when you have stretched to your fullest.

3. Exhale and try to sink lower into your stretch.

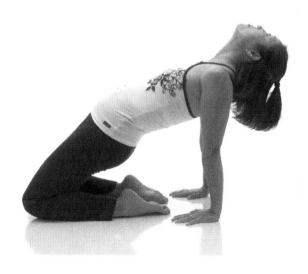

Time To Get Down
To Business
9am – 11am Spleen Meridian Time

Spleen meridian time is when you are just starting the workday and should focus on the most difficult tasks of the day.

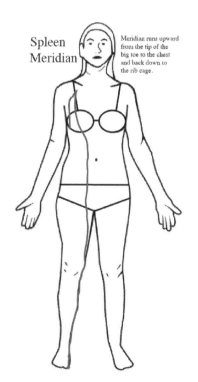

Spleen Meridian

Meridian runs upward from the tip of the big toe to the chest and back down to the rib cage.

Spleen chi is directly related to a person's body weight and muscle tone. If spleen chi is deficient then you will lack muscle tone and have extra weight on your body. If your spleen chi is strong and vibrant you will be healthy.

The Journal Of Clinical Nursing (Volume 17, Issue 9, pages 1174–1181, May 2008) reported in April 2008 that in a double blind study of premature babies showed that massaging the stomach, spleen and bladder meridians helped premature infants gain weight. Here is their stated conclusion:

"An experimental trial established the effects of using acupressure and meridian massage on increasing body weight in premature infants. Acupressure and meridian massage have a significant effect on weight gain in premature infants."

So, before buying the latest diet pills and exercise gadgets try working on your spleen meridian chi.

According to Traditional Chinese Medicine you can support the spleen meridian by wearing yellow clothing or jewelry, and by singing.

The best way to enhance your chi at this time is to work hard at the tasks at hand. Get out your list and start working.

Makko-ho Stomach and Spleen Meridian Stretch:

See stretch in the previous chapter.

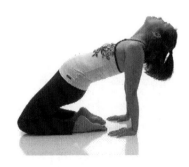

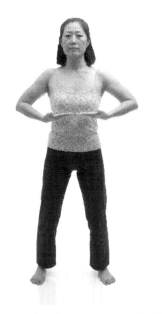

Stomach and Spleen Chi Kung:

1) Stand naturally upright. Sink your chi down through your feet and grip the center of the earth and grip the ground with your toes.

2) Inhale and bring your hands to your solar plexus just below the middle of your chest, with your palms facing up and fingers pointing at each other feel the chi in your palms.

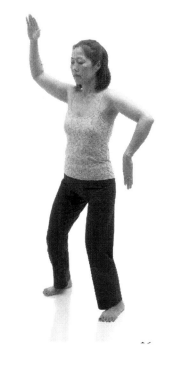

3) Exhale and rotate your right palm away from your body and up, and rotate your left palm toward your body and down; extend both hands up and down.

4) Now inhale and bring both hands down

facing each other at your solar plexus.

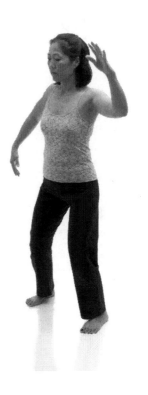

5) Now rotate your left palm out away from your body and up, and rotate your right palm in towards your body and down. Then extend both palms up and down and exhale as you did on the first time. Repeat for a total of 6 inhalations and exhalations.

Joy and Meaning at High Noon
11am – 1pm Heart Meridian Time

At heart meridian time (11am - 1pm) you tackled the toughest tasks of your day for the last two hours and now it is time to switch gears and work on the tasks that are productive and give you joy and meaning.

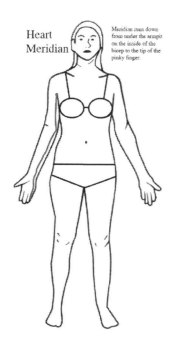

Heart Meridian

Meridian runs down from under the armpit on the inside of the bicep to the tip of the pinky finger.

Your yang energy is about to peak at noon and switch over to your yin energy at 1pm setting up the rest of the day as a time to start to slow down and complete a good day's work.

The Institute of HeartMath an internationally recognized nonprofit research and education organization dedicated to heart-based living has been conducting scientific studies on the heart and its relationship to the entire body and specific organs. Here is what they have to say about the heart, "Our research and that of others indicate that the heart is far more than a simple pump.

The heart is, in fact, a highly complex, self-organized information processing center with its own functional "brain" that communicates with and influences the cranial brain via the nervous system, hormonal system and other pathways. These influences profoundly affect brain function and most of the body's major organs, and ultimately determine the quality of life."

The Institute of HeartMath is using modern day scientific techniques to prove what Traditional Chinese Medicine has known for thousands of years; that the heart is the Emperor of the body! It is believed to be the home of our consciousness and intelligence and that it rules over our entire body.

According to Traditional Chinese Medicine you can support the heart meridian by wearing red, laughing and pursuing activities that give you joy.

> *The best way to enhance your chi at this time of day is through expressive, joyful productive activities.*

Makko-ho Heart and Small Intestine Stretch:

This stretch will bring your emotions into balance and give you a feeling of being centered and calm. Sit on the floor and place the soles of your feet together, and bring them back as far as comfortable to the groin.

Exhale while clasping your feet with your hands and relax your head forward with your arms resting on your legs. Try to keep your shoulders relaxed. Take 3-4 breaths in this position and with each exhale relax your knees a little further to the floor. Only go as far as you can without straining.

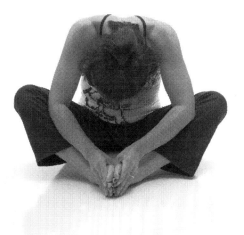

Start to Slow Your Pace
1pm – 3pm
Small Intestine Meridian Time

At Small intestine meridian time you are moving more toward yin energy. You can take a step back here and slow down a bit. This is not a time to tackle tough assignments.

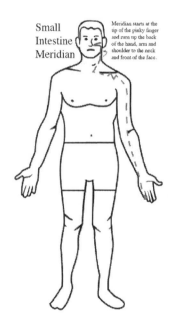

Yang energy will still be carrying you forward but do not tackle really tough problems at this time of day.

According to Traditional Chinese Medicine you can support the small intestine meridian by wearing red.

The best way to enhance your chi at this time is to eat a healthy relaxing lunch and start slowing your day down a bit.

Makko-ho Heart and Small Intestine Stretch:
See stretch in the previous chapter Heart Meridian time.

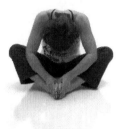

Small Intestine 5 Acupressure Point:

Small Intestine 5 (SI5) improves concentration and clarity of mind. Located on the topside of wrist, in line with the pinky and just above the bony protrusion of the wrist.

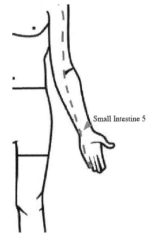

Small Intestine 5

To find SI5 measure one finger width below the crease of the wrist, it will be in the depression right above the bony protrusion. Remember it is in line with the pinky not the bony protrusion of the wrist. Press on this point improves concentration and helps with the clarity of your mind to make better decisions.

The 4 O'clock Office Blues
3pm – 5pm Bladder Meridian Time

At Bladder meridian time (3pm - 5pm) it is best to start planning the end of your work day by wrapping up minor details and to start mentally preparing evening pursuits.

Save this time of day for doing busy work like filing, reviewing documents, returning phone calls, and sending emails.

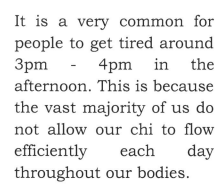

Bladder Meridian

Meridian starts at the eye socket, over the top of the head and runs behind neck and down back of the body to the tip of the little toe.

It is a very common for people to get tired around 3pm - 4pm in the afternoon. This is because the vast majority of us do not allow our chi to flow efficiently each day throughout our bodies.

We stay up too late, we don't exercise between 5am-7am, we don't eat

27

breakfast at stomach meridian time, and we eat a hurried lunch at small intestine time and get right back to work. This leads to a crash of energy system at this time and the need for most people to reach for coffee, chocolate, or some sugary treat to try and boost their energy level.

Of course, this only leads to temporary boost and a crash of energy and then we drag our-selves home from work more tired than when we left in the morning.

As this cycle of ignoring our energy flow continues, day in and day out for years disease and illness have the perfect opportunity to develop.

According to Traditional Chinese Medicine you can support the bladder meridian by wearing blue.

> *The best way to enhance your chi at this time is to slow down and take care of all the menial tasks that need to be done for the day.*

Makko-ho Bladder and Kidney Stretch:

This stretch will open up the bladder meridian that runs down your neck, back and legs. Sit on the floor or your mat and straighten your legs out in front of you and point your toes to the sky. You can adjust your position by grabbing under each of your buttocks and pulling out from under you to give you firmer seating. As you inhale bring your arms straight above your head with your biceps close to your ears. Ex-hale, fold your torso over your legs while stretching with your arms to grab your over the top of your toes. If you can reach your kidney wellspring point just be-low the balls of your feet you can press on it. If not, do not strain yourself and just send your thoughts of wellness to this point. Breath in for 3 - 4 counts and sink lower into the stretch if you can. Repeat 3 - 4 times.

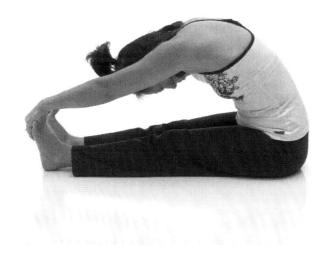

Relax By Candlelight
5pm – 7pm Kidney Meridian Time

Kidney meridian time (5pm - 7pm) is all about switching from the fast paced yang energy of the day to the mellow yin energy of the evening. This will help your body restore itself while you sleep.

This is the time of day when the sun is setting and the daytime is relinquishing to nighttime.

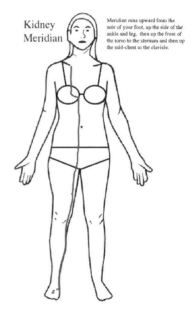

Kidney Meridian

Meridian runs upward from the sole of your foot, up the side of the ankle and leg, then up the front of the torso to the sternum and then up the mid-chest to the clavicle.

Inside your body yang energy is setting and yin energy is rising but only if you let it.

Many illnesses are caused by people not allowing yin energy to take over while they continually press on with the day's work and allow yang energy to flow uninterrupted.

If you're are not living as close as you can to the natural chi cycle then it is very easy to continue to push your-self through kidney meridian time. In our westernized culture we are as far removed from our natural energy cycle as can be.

As mentioned earlier one of the main causes of this is electricity and what it powers; lights, television and computers. Less than 100 years ago electricity and lights were not available and we followed the natural cycle of the sun much more closely. Rising early with the sun and going to bed early when the sun set.

In the early 1900's most people slept 10 hours a night and their bodies were well rested because the chi cycle could complete its work. It will be very important in pericardium meridian time (7pm - 9pm) that you keep your use of lights, television, computers and anything that emits light to a minimum.

The longer you leave the lights on the longer you are fooling your body that it is daytime. Turn off the "electric" lights and try talking, reading, and relaxing by candlelight.

According to Traditional Chinese Medicine you can support the kidney meridian by wearing blue.

> *The best way to enhance your chi at this time is to perform activities that help your body switch from the use of yang to yin energy.*

This can be achieved by spending time with family, friends or a lover (by candlelight!). At this time any activity that helps you relax is helpful.

Makko-ho Bladder and Kidney Stretch:

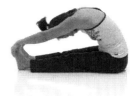

See Previous Chapter

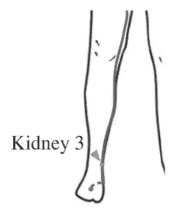

Kidney 3

Kidney 3 is beneficial for emotional well-being and is located on the inside of the foot, halfway between the Achilles tendon and the side of the anklebone.

You can press this point with a finger or the tip of a pencil eraser. It has a healing effect when there is too much fear in the body and it has been said to help with lower back pain.

Guard Yourself Against Technology
7pm – 9pm Pericardium Meridian Time

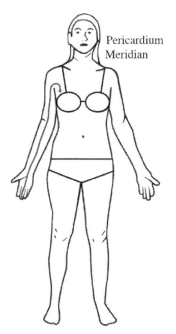

Pericardium Meridian

Pericardium meridian time (7pm - 9pm) is an extremely crucial time in the 24-hour cycle of chi. The pericardium is the thin membrane that surrounds the heart and the roots of the great blood vessels. In Traditional Chinese Medicine it is the protector of the heart.

This is the time of day when you must prepare to go to sleep in the next few hours and must be careful not to allow today's modern conveniences of light, television, e-book readers, smart phones and computers to distract you from your natural instinct to go to sleep early.

Once you stay up too late you cannot get up early and begin the day in colon meridian time (5am - 7am). In today's modern world we have lost touch with our natural surroundings and the natural cycle of life. Electricity, and more specifically light, has helped human beings control our environment and kept us safe but it has also hurt us by moving us further away from nature.

In the book, *Lights Out: Sleep, Sugar and Survival* , T.S. Wiley and Bent Formby state, "the disastrous slide in the health of the American people corresponds to the increase in light-generating night activities and the carbohydrate consumption that follows." They argue (backed up by 100's of scientific studies) that not sleeping a recommended 9.5 hrs in the winter (September 15th - April 15th) as we would if we were in touch with the natural cycle of the sun; leads to obesity, diabetes, heart disease, and cancer.

Traditional Chinese Medicine has instinctively known this for thousands of years but it has taken a healthcare crisis for western medicine to start to wonder what the causes may be.

If you were going to wake up at 6am then you would need to be asleep (not reading a book or watching TV in bed) at 9:00pm. So you would want to start getting ready for bed at 8:00pm and be in bed by 8:30pm in order to be asleep at 9:00pm.

According to Traditional Chinese Medicine you can support the Pericardium meridian by wearing red.

The best way to enhance your chi at this time before you go to sleep to do things you enjoy most in life (reading, music, crafts or hobbies) and then get ready for bed.

Makko-ho Pericardium and Triple Heater Stretch:

This stretch opens up the two meridians that are responsible for protecting the heart and for balancing our emotional state. Sit on the floor, cross your legs and arms with each hand touching the opposite knee. Take a breath in and relax the upper body forward with your elbows drifting toward the floor. Breathe in for 3 - 4 counts and sink lower into the stretch if you can. Repeat 3 - 4 times. Now reverse the crossing of your legs and arms and repeat.

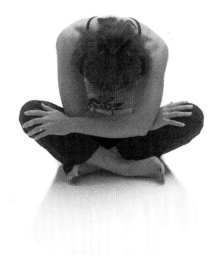

Fire In The Hole
9pm – 11pm Triple Heater
Meridian Time

Triple heater meridian time (9pm - 11pm) is the beginning of our sleep cycle and everything we have done from 5pm until now should have prepared us to go to bed and fall asleep easily and comfortably.

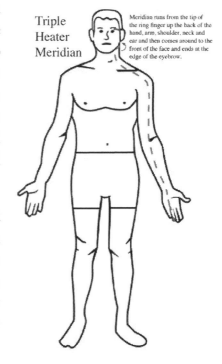

Triple Heater Meridian

Meridian runs from the tip of the ring finger up the back of the hand, arm, shoulder, neck and ear and then comes around to the front of the face and ends at the edge of the eyebrow.

The Triple Heater is not an organ by western medical standards. It is the combination of three areas of the body responsible for our metabolism.

The Upper Burners (Lungs and Heart), Middle Burners (Stomach, Pancreas, Liver), and Lower Burners (Intestines, Kidneys, Bladder).

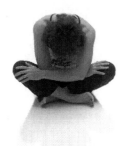

Makko-ho Pericardium and Triple Heater Stretch:

See previous chapter for this stretch.

The best way to enhance your chi at this time is to be falling asleep

Triple Heater Acupressure Point:

In his book, *The Healing Power of Acupressure and Acupuncture: A Complete Guide to Timeless Traditions and Modern Practices*, author Matthew D. Bauer suggests to use Triple Heater 5 in conjunction with Pericardium 6 for a balancing of yin and yang.

Triple Heater 5 is on top of the forearm three finger lengths above the wrist and Pericardium 6 is directly below it on the underside of the forearm.

You can use your thumb to press one point and the tip of your index finger and your middle ringer to press the other point at the same time. Hold for 30 seconds while breathing deeply and repeat.

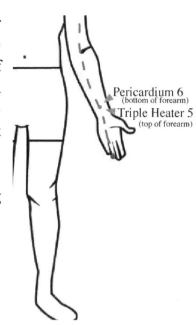

Pericardium 6
(bottom of forearm)

Triple Heater 5
(top of forearm)

Sleep, Sleep, Sleep
11pm – 1am Gall Bladder
Meridian Time

Gall bladder meridian time (11pm - 1am) is a crucial time to be asleep. There are many biological functions that take place during this time (your first hours of sleep) to restore the body and mind. Gall bladder meridian time can be a very important time to practice chi kung for advance practitioners.

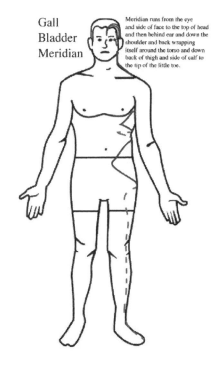

Gall Bladder Meridian

Meridian runs from the eye and side of face to the top of head and then behind ear and down the shoulder and back wrapping itself around the torso and down back of thigh and side of calf to the tip of the little toe.

However, for beginning students it is best to practice chi kung upon waking, during lunch hour or before sleep until they are more skilled at chi kung.

According to Traditional Chinese Medicine you can support the gall bladder meridian by wearing green.

> *The best way to enhance your chi at this time is to be fast asleep.*

Makko-ho Gall Bladder and Liver Stretch:

This stretch opens and balances this pair of meridians. Sit on the floor, spread your legs out wide, and flex your toes up. With your back straight turn your torso in line with your left foot and bring your left arm over your left ear. Rest your right arm wherever comfortable. Bend your torso sideways toward your left foot while keep-ing your buttocks firmly and evenly pressed to the floor. Breath and try to sink lower into the position with each exhale. Repeat 3 -5 times. Do not strain. Your body will guide you as to how far it can go. Repeat on the opposite side with your right arm.

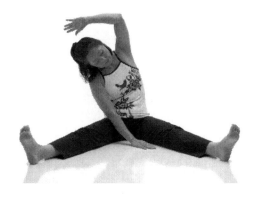

A Crucial Time For Repair
1am – 3am Liver Meridian Time

Liver meridian time (1:00am - 3:00am) is a crucial time to be asleep so that your liver can perform

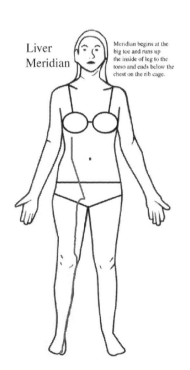

Liver Meridian

Meridian begins at the big toe and runs up the inside of leg to the torso and ends below the chest on the rib cage.

many metabolic functions to keep your body healthy and in homeostasis. If you find yourself awake at this time it may because you have eaten a meal high in fat or had too many alcoholic drinks earlier in the evening and now your liver is having trouble processing all that fat and/or alcohol.

If your lifestyle and diet have not been

very healthy up until now you may have a fatty liver that is sluggish and not functioning at its peak.

One of the principles of chi flow through the meridians is that it will be at a peak and a low within the 24hr period. When the liver chi is flowing at its peak the small intestine chi (1pm -3pm) is at its lowest point of the cycle of chi. This is one reason it is best not to eat late at night before bed. This combined with the possibility of compromised liver will certainly keep you up at night.

According to Traditional Chinese Medicine you can support the Liver meridian by wearing green.

The best way to enhance your chi at this time is to be fast asleep.

Liver 2 Acupressure Point:

Liver 2 can be used to reduce the body of anger. Be-cause you are reducing anger rotate the point counter clockwise when pressing.

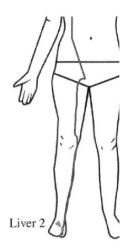

You can locate Liver 2 in between the webbing connecting the big toe and the second toe.

Liver 2

It is said to use this point only when there is heat, as when you're red in the face or your skin feels hot to the touch and you're feeling warm from prolonged anger (not from exertion). Don't use when weak or low on energy.

Makko-ho Gall Bladder and Liver Stretch:

See previous chapter.

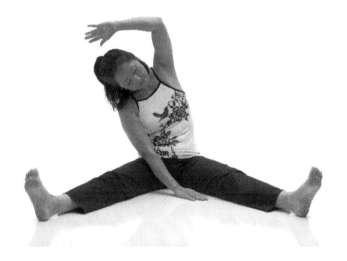

Resources

For more information on our iPhone App for the and chi enhancing exercises please visit our website at:

www.BodyEnergyBook.com

Contact the Author:

Matthew Harrigan

Email: bodyenergybooks@gmail.com

Made in the USA
Columbia, SC
23 December 2020

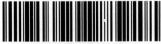